AMAZING

‖‖‖‖‖‖‖‖‖‖‖‖‖‖‖
MW01539271

Mother of All Anti-Oxidants to Live Longer and Healthy

By: Prem Chhatwani

Table of Contents

Preface

Over the years I had lot of interest in Alternate Therapies, including Homoeopathic medicines and Herbal and Ayurvedic treatments for various diseases.

At age 28 I got hit by Asthma. My Dad had Asthma and his younger brother (my uncle) had Asthma as well. My grandmother, father side, also had suffered from Asthma.

So I kind of inherited the disease but at a later age than as a child.

My Mom had heart problems but she actually died of Cancer in her late fifties.

With family history like that, I did not know what to expect in my older years. At age of around 50, with slightly high Cholesterol (230-240) and still using inhalers like Albuterol Sulfate and Cortisone (Prednisone) pills very frequently for my Asthma, I ran across some books and publications that opened my mind to try alternate remedies.

1) I started drinking Magnetized water every day as there were no side effects or interaction with my drugs for Asthma. One thing I must

say Asthma patients should drink more water. Keep the body hydrated. The benefits of drinking magnetized water are realized very slowly but it also helps heart and lungs. It basically removes deposits from arteries and air passages in the lungs. Mind you, western medicine does not recognize this. Benefits of magnetized water would be another kindle book. If interested check this link but not required at all.
http://www.amazon.com/dp/B007IO7DN8

Or simply email me at pjan86@gmail.com for a free report on this.

By Age 60 I was completely free from Asthma. Now I cannot prove Magnetized water did it. You the reader decide and investigate and be the judge. Main stream medical practitioners will make a fun of this. I got off my inhalers and Prednisone Cortisone pills which by the way affect bone density. I slowly improved my bone density with exercise, Calcium and Vitamin D.

2) I investigated Chelation Therapy. I found a certified Doctor, M.D. then in our small town in Ohio (USA). She was certified to do the procedure of administering by IV EDTA

(Ethylene Diamine Tetra Acetic acid) compound, approved by FDA for lead toxicity. I could see her clinic full of patients hooked up IV rigs on wheels, reading books or working on their paper work. It was sight to be seen.

I decided to take two treatments a week, for six weeks. I never did consult my primary physician. I felt safe taking the treatment as a precaution to avoid heart problems in the future due to family history. I also had personal interest to see how it feels so that I can tell others my own experience. Once again I cannot recommend anything. There are several books on the subject. You can also read my Kindle book here: **http://tinyurl.com/n7r7ge6**

The best part now is that at age 75 I have no Asthma and my heart is healthy but I do take small dose of prescribed medicine for cholesterol to keep it under control. I do consume red meat, fish and drink red wine. I am seriously considering taking additional few Chelation treatments to help clean up my arteries as a precaution. I will consult an approved doctor trained and certified by ACAM for Chelation.

Let us now get back to main topic of this book "Glutathione".

1. Introduction

Glutathione, also known as GSH, is the protector and detoxifier of your body's cells. Produced by every cell in your body, glutathione is your first line of defense against toxins, radiation, heavy metals, oxidative stress and accelerated aging. Glutathione helps protect the DNA in your cells and supports your immune system as well as the rapid proliferation of immune cells. It is your body's Master Antioxidant, because it deals with all forms of oxidation and has the ability to recycle itself. It also recycles other antioxidants such as Vitamin C and alpha Lipoic acid.

Modern research has shown that individuals who have low levels of glutathione have a high association with illness. Unfortunately, decreased levels of glutathione can be brought about by continual stress upon the immune system. This is a ferocious cycle. While you need glutathione for a productive immune system, a weakened immune system hampers the production of glutathione. Various daily activities can also reduce your glutathione levels such as stress, exercise, infection, injury, poor diet, and environmental toxins. Your glutathione, or in other words, your body's natural defense against aging and cellular damage starts to decline as you age, decreasing by about 10% to 15% every decade!

It is amazing I have been going to my primary physician at least twice a year to check my blood profile and keep track of my health and so on. In all these 70+ years none of the doctors have mentioned anything about Glutathione levels in my blood and its vital role in keeping good health.

So in my last visit I asked my doctor if he will recommend blood test for glutathione levels. His reply was that it is not required and neither will insurance cover the test. He did say that I can take glutathione as a supplement and it does not require any prescription. I did not explore further with him on this topic.

I have also been going regularly to my natural health practitioner. He is M.D. but promotes natural health therapies. I go there for my regular EDTA Chelation therapy to maintain healthy heart and blood circulation. However he never did mention anything about glutathione, either. So I finally asked him and found out that he does offer glutathione treatments intravenously. I plan to pursue that Treatment with him shortly after I am done using glutathione patches.

I practice what I preach or write about to be more realistic to my readers in expressing my own experience.

It appears that there is a growing awareness about this master anti-oxidant now and people like me are seeking out how to best use this very important health supplement. I am also trying to make other health conscious individuals like you aware of this wonderful supplement. It may help you or someone you know.

One of the best ways to determine whether you would be ready to use glutathione, the master anti-oxidant, is to contemplate these questions: Do you have metal toxicity? Your regular blood test will not do the justice in finding out this. You find a doctor who is trained and possibly certified to do Chelations. He will then do a challenge test with compound called EDTA for metal toxicity. This is done intravenously (I V drip) in doctor's office. Then urine sample is collected over 24 hours.

The sample of that urine is then sent to a certified Lab. to check levels of common metals like Aluminum, Cadmium, Lead, and so on.

Do you suffer from Physical stress?
You should know the answer.

Do you have cardiovascular, lung, digestive and kidney disorders?
Your medical tests will establish this.

Ideally, your reply to the questions was "yes". Those characteristics are typical among individuals who use glutathione-the master anti-oxidant. You have promptly taken the first step towards using glutathione!

2. What is Glutathione?

Glutathione is a substance produced naturally by the liver. It is also found in fruits, vegetables, and meats.

Glutathione is made up of 3 amino acids, glycine, glutamic acid and cysteine. Glycine and glutamic acid are both readily available in abundance in much of the food we eat. Cysteine is much harder for the body to come by, making it the limiting factor for glutathione production.

Glutathione has been called the Mother of all antioxidants as it's said to prevent aging, cancer, heart disease, dementia and more, and necessary to treat everything from autism to Alzheimer's disease. Our bodies when working correctly and with a good nutritious diet, produce glutathione by itself but several things lessen this action. A poor diet, pollution, toxins, medications, stress, trauma, aging, infections and radiation all deplete the glutathione in our systems, and these days, we sure have enough of all that.

Listen to Dr. OZ

https://www.youtube.com/watch?feature=player embedded&v=S0l_4_DP5Rw

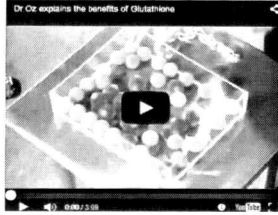

Also listen to Mark Hyman, MD. Please be patient and listen.

https://www.youtube.com/watch?v=Eh2PYQB ICWs

3. Benefits of Increased levels of Glutathione

Increasing your Glutathione level will naturally increase your energy, detoxify your body and significantly strengthen your immune system.

Glutathione provides many benefits to the human body. People with higher glutathione levels have been found to experience:

- Reduced joint discomfort and inflammation
- Strengthened immune systems
- Improved stamina and endurance
- Faster recovery from exercise
- Greater mental clarity and focus
- More restful sleep
- Reduced anxiety and depression
- Help with Parkinson disease and Alzheimer's.
- Anti –allergenic
- Help with glaucoma and Cataracts
- Anti-cancer

- Avoid kidney disorders
- Reduces blood fat and helps with obesity
- Great booster for our immune system
- Excellent detoxifier
- Protects against viral infections

4. How to Improve Your Glutathione Levels and Live Healthy and Longer!

Even though scientists have proclaimed glutathione as the most important antioxidant in your body, they've had one heck of a time actually increasing it in your body.

You see, as you age your body becomes less and less efficient at recycling and producing glutathione.

And since glutathione is the antioxidant which controls all other antioxidants - you start aging! The faster your glutathione levels drop, the faster you age...it's as simple as that.

And to make matters worse - as you age your body starts to encounter even MORE stresses and free radicals than it did when you were in your 20's.

Effectively enhancing glutathione levels through oral supplementation can be a bit tricky. The problem with most glutathione supplements is the fact that both reduced glutathione and glutathione disulfide are quickly broken down during the digestive process. Destroying the glutathione molecule and allowing only a small fraction of the ingested glutathione to be absorbed intact.

Supplementing with **Glutathione** in the past has been difficult and remains difficult, as scientific research shows that **Glutathione** taken orally is **NOT** well absorbed across the GI tract.

Liposomal glutathione and Acetyl glutathione supplements offer a far more bioavailable form of our master antioxidant. Both of these protect the glutathione molecule from damage throughout the digestive process, ensuring optimal absorption of intact glutathione for maximum health benefits.

Liposomal Glutathione Explained

As already mentioned, glutathione molecules rapidly degrade during the digestive process. Using liposomal glutathione is one way to overcome this problem. A liposome is an artificial vesicle consisting of an aqueous (water) core and it is enclosed in one or more phospholipid layer. By encapsulating the glutathione molecule in this phospholipid structure, it protects the GSH during the digestive process.

The downfall of liposomal glutathione supplements is the fact that over time this phospholipid shield begins to break down the glutathione molecule. If the supplement sits on a shelf for too long, or for any reason is not delivered to the end user in a timely manner it becomes increasingly ineffective. When looking for liposomal glutathione supplements it is extremely important to ensure the supplement is fresh and used promptly in order to achieve the best results.

Acetyl Glutathione Explained

Acetylation is commonly used in organic and pharmaceutical chemistry, one acetylated drug that almost everyone recognizes is acetylsalicylic acid (aspirin). When an acetyl group is bonded to an organic molecule its ability to cross the selectively permeable blood-brain barrier increases. This increases the effect of the organic molecule and the intensity of these effects.

When the glutathione molecule is acetylated it is rapidly absorbed by the body, ensuring the GSH is absorbed intact. Offering a far more bioavailable option for supplementing glutathione levels. Acetyl glutathione differs from liposomal glutathione because it does not have the same problem with shelf-life. Acetyl glutathione will stay intact and retain its molecular integrity far longer than liposomal glutathione. This makes acetyl glutathione the best option for directly enhancing usable GSH levels.

Just Remember to take prescribed dose regularly. You will experience better results. Furthermore, you will experience detoxifying effect of glutathione, especially when the day comes to actually use glutathione-the master anti-oxidant.

Also drink plenty of water. This is definitely an ideal rule to follow. This will improve detoxification process.

5. Glutathione Enhancing Supplements

Glutathione precursors are nutrients that provide the building blocks for glutathione production in the body. Other nutrients have the ability to enhance the recycling process of glutathione, increasing the amount of glutathione reductase. By incorporating both precursors and natural glutathione recyclers you can significantly enhance GSH levels without directly supplementing glutathione. We highlight a few of the most potent glutathione enhancing supplements and precursors below. Here is a short list of some more nutritional supplements that have been shown to improve glutathione levels in the body: Vitamins E and C, Selenium, Silymarin (milk thistle), Magnesium and Zinc.

N-acetyl cysteine

As described earlier Glutathione is made up of 3 amino acids, glycine, glutamic acid and cysteine. Glycine and glutamic acid are both readily available in abundance in much of the food we eat. Cysteine is much harder for the body to come by, making it the rate limiting factor for glutathione production.

A derivative of cysteine, which is a direct precursor and limiting factor in glutathione synthesis, N-acetyl cysteine (NAC) yields nearly as many health benefits as glutathione itself.

N-acetyl cysteine is commonly used to treat acetaminophen overdoses and as a mucolytic agent. With powerful antioxidant properties all its own, NAC is one of the most effective ways to enhance endogenous glutathione synthesis.

By enhancing cysteine levels in the body through orally supplementing N-acetyl cysteine, you can improve GSH production immensely for a short period of time. Making it important to supplement regularly if you intend on maintaining high GSH levels solely through NAC supplements.

Some of the foods that contain precursors, such as cysteine, include poultry, wheat, broccoli, eggs, garlic, capsicum, red meat, fish, dairy products, beans, fruits, vegetables, asparagus, avocado and walnuts.

R-Alpha Lipoic Acid.

Alpha Lipoic acid is a remarkable antioxidant, partially due to the fact that it is both water soluble and fat soluble. This grants this antioxidant a VIP pass through the body and its systems, passing effortlessly through the blood-brain barrier and other selectively permeable membranes.

Lipoic acid helps protect against oxidative stress generated by high glucose levels. Alpha-Lipoic acid consists of two different forms (isomers) that have vastly different properties.

The "R" form is the biologically active component (native to the body) that is responsible for Lipoic acid's phenomenal antioxidant effect.

The "S" form is produced from chemical manufacture and is not very biologically active. Typical alpha-Lipoic acid supplements consist of the "R" and "S" form in a 50/50 ratio. That means a 100 mg alpha-Lipoic acid supplement is providing 50 mg of the biologically active "R" form.

The human body normally produces and uses the "R" form of Lipoic acid. This active form, **R-Lipoic acid**, significantly supports healthy inflammatory response, is a potent free-radical scavenger and has been shown to be more potent than the combined "R" and "S" forms that comprise most alpha-Lipoic acid supplements.

Also there is **Super R-Lipoic Acid** supplement available. This has demonstrated superior bioavailability, stability, and potency for a variety of health benefits. This breakthrough converts the biologically active "R" form of Lipoic acid to sodium-R-Lipoic acid, which, in a recent human study achieved **10–30 times** higher peak blood levels than pure R-Lipoic acid. Not only does this newer Lipoic acid formulation reach higher peak blood levels, it also achieves them sooner, ensuring rapid uptake from the plasma into the tissues. A recent study showed that oral ingestion of Super R-Lipoic Acid reached peak plasma concentrations within just **10–20 minutes** of supplementation. This is available from a company in USA called Life Extension.

I personally take 1 cap. 240mg. first thing in the morning as my daily dose.

The superior antioxidant effects of R-Lipoic acid are already well known for supporting healthy mitochondrial function. Now, Super R-Lipoic Acid provides even more potent benefits for preserving youthful cellular energy levels.

ALA. Both alpha Lipoic acid and R-alpha Lipoic acid offer immense health benefits but R-ALA is only found in the highest quality nutritional supplements. It is more expensive, but far more effective in comparable doses. R-ALA increases glutathione synthesis by increasing the expression of gamma-glutamyl cysteine ligase (GCL), the rate limiting factor in glutathione synthesis. It also increases the cellular uptake of cysteine, one of the fundamental building blocks for endogenous glutathione production.

One of the most beneficial effects of alpha-Lipoic acid is its ability to regenerate other essential antioxidants such as vitamins C and E, coenzyme Q10, and glutathione, and the activities of superoxide dismutase (SOD) and glutathione peroxidase (GPx). The evidence is especially strong for the ability of DHLA (dihydrolipoic acid, a reduced form of alpha-Lipoic acid) to recycle vitamin E. This is apparently achieved directly by quenching tocopherol radicals or indirectly by reducing vitamin C or increasing the levels of ubiquinol (a derivative of CoQ10) and glutathione, that, in turn, helps regenerate tissue levels of vitamin E.

The best natural way to raise your glutathione levels is to eat more vegetables, nuts, fresh fruits, poultry and fish. These are the basics of the Mediterranean diet, which is proven to prevent dementia.

But even people who eat well often get only half the glutathione they really need.

The answer is a glutathione supplement, but here's where you have to be careful because most are poorly absorbed. Look for a form called Setria, which can be easily absorbed by your body and is proven to raise glutathione levels as suggested by Mark Stengler, MD. He recommends 1,000 mg per day for most people. Review this site for valuable information http://setriaglutathione.com/about

Get to know Immunocal.
Immunocal is an all-natural non-prescription health product available worldwide. This special protein holds many national and international patents and is medically recognized in the Physicians' Desk Reference ("PDR" U.S.A.) and Compendium of Pharmaceutical Specialties ("CPS" Canada). It has undergone over 30 years of research and has been taken safely and effectively by millions of individuals.

Immunocal acts in two ways – it is a very high quality protein that provides all the amino acids your body needs, and more critically, it raises levels of "glutathione" in our body. Immunocal contains specific fragile proteins that supply your body with the building blocks needed for the production of *glutathione* in your cells. These building blocks are called "precursors" and glutathione precursors are relatively rare in our normal diets. Unfortunately, eating glutathione does not effectively raise glutathione in the cells; this is why we need the precursors.

There have been no known harmful side effects of using Immunocal or any other Immunotec product while on medications. However, to be safe, it is better to consult your physician, if you have any questions.

As a natural source of the glutathione precursor for the maintenance of the good health, 10 grams per day (one pouch) of cysteine is recommended. However for the maintenance of a strong immune system, 20 grams per day is recommended (two pouches). Clinical trials in patients with AIDS, chronic obstructive pulmonary disease (COPD), cancer and chronic fatigue syndrome have used 30 - 40 grams per day without ill effect.

Immunocal is best administered on an empty stomach or with a light meal. Concomitant intake of another high protein load may adversely affect absorption.

Who should avoid Immunocal?

People who have a specific allergy to milk proteins (this is different from lactose intolerance) need to avoid this product. People who are taking immunosuppressive medication in the case of organ transplants should not take this product.

Who should be cautious with Immunocal?

People who are on a protein-restricted diet need to calculate into their daily equation 9 grams of protein per pouch and should not exceed their daily protein limit. Keep in mind that Immunocal has a very high "biological value" as a protein and will supply an excellent source of amino acids for those individuals who may be challenged nutritionally.

Are there any side effects and what to do?

Abdominal cramps and bloating can occasionally occur. This is usually corrected by increasing your fluid intake. Rarely, some individuals may experience a rash with this product. Although this may indicate an allergy, it may represent a "detoxification reaction". In both cases, discontinuing the product should resolve the symptom. If any symptoms are severe or persistent, contact your health care practitioner.

Is Immunocal safe to take with medication?

There have been no known harmful side effects of using Immunocal or any other Immunotec product while on medications. However, to be safe, please consult with your physician if you have any concerns.

How to take Glutathione

People take glutathione by mouth for treating cataracts and glaucoma, preventing aging, treating or preventing alcoholism, asthma, cancer, heart disease (atherosclerosis and high cholesterol), hepatitis, liver disease, diseases that weaken the body's defense system (including AIDS and chronic fatigue syndrome), memory loss, Alzheimer's disease, osteoarthritis, and Parkinson's disease. Glutathione is also used for maintaining the body's defense system (immune system) and fighting   metal toxicity and drug poisoning.

Glutathione is breathed in (inhaled) for treating lung diseases, including idiopathic pulmonary fibrosis, cystic fibrosis, and lung disease in people with HIV disease.

Healthcare providers give glutathione as a shot (by injection into the muscle) for preventing poisonous side effects of cancer treatment (chemotherapy) and for treating the inability to father a child   (male infertility).

Healthcare providers also give glutathione intravenously (by injection into the vein, by IV) for preventing "tired blood" (anemia) in kidney patients undergoing hemodialysis treatment, preventing kidney problems after heart bypass surgery, treating Parkinson's disease, improving blood flow and decreasing clotting in individuals with "hardening of the arteries" (atherosclerosis), treating diabetes, and preventing toxic side effects of chemotherapy.

Glutathione is also available as a patch. It has much better absorption rate than oral supplements.
If you live in USA you can buy oral supplement called "Glutathione Plus" from Bel Marra Health 1-800-531-0466. I have no association with them. I have been using this product as well as Patches mentioned above.
Also Max International, an MLM company offers a similar product called "MaxGXL"
www.max.com
Please be advised I have no association with any of these suppliers. I prefer intravenous delivery being most effective, then next the patches and finally the oral supplements. Some

supplements are better than others. Do your research. Also read testimonials for general guidance.

7. Testimonials

Reviewer: 45-54 Male on Treatment for 1 to 6 months

I began receiving IV treatments from my doctor as part of a weight loss and health routine. I should also note that I have changed my diet and exercise plan. I lost a substantial amount of weight the first 30 days - 28 lbs. to be exact. Month three of my treatment I became very ill, flu like symptoms, I almost thought I had food poising. It last three days. Two weeks later I became ill again, same symptoms. I called my Doctor and asked if it was possible for the Glutathione IV to give me this reaction, he said; "Glutathione can cause a loss of Zinc, you should take Zinc". I took zinc lozenges and after 12 hours felt better. I don't know if anyone else has experienced this. I do know that I am normally very healthy and do not get the cold or flu.

Reviewer: Nancy Mac, 65-74 Female on Treatment for less than 1 month.

I took 250 mg orally once a day to reduce inflammation in knuckles due to arthritis. Within TWO DAYS 4 of the 8 knuckles on the back of my hand had FLATTENED, the other 4 are taking a little longer. It is a miracle. Also my brown spots are lightening. I can hardly wait to see what else it will do.

Reviewer: 35-44 Female on Treatment for less than 1 month.
I am hypothyroid and it had given me more energy and overall I feel better.

Reviewer: 55-64 Female on Treatment for 1 to less than 2 years.

Highly effective for skin care. Used for one year, can see a big difference in skin color. The complements keep coming. Easy to use.

Reviewer: Stephanie, 55-64 Female on Treatment for 1 to 6 months.

Skin pores in my face had decreased and waiting that it will all disappear, redness in my chest I described as burn from sun had disappeared, I am waiting that my skin will get lighter.

Reviewer: Tseely, 45-54 Female on Treatment for 1 to 6 months.

It has most certainly boosted my immunity. I believe my overall appearance of my skin has improved.

Reviewer: 35-44 Male on Treatment for 1 to 6 months.

I was diagnosed with osteoarthritis and could not weight train the same as I used to. After taking glutathione for 30 days, my dumb bell bench press increased from 40kg to 55kg and there were no more symptoms of osteoarthritis. It really works.

57 years old women:

I am probably more sensitive to changes in my body than the average person, but the evening after taking the first capsule of glutathione that afternoon, I was lying in bed and felt my legs feel fuller as though the circulation was in full force for the first time in years. After a week of taking one capsule a day, I went for a walk on a cold, wet evening, and for the first time in years,

I experienced no leg cramps. Great stuff that I will take from now on.

smulic (Parkinson's Disease)
I am amazed at how much it's helping me with my energy and tremors

Theta1 (Parkinson's Disease)
My experience with Glutathione....before my treatment I could not walk to the Mail box and back…after one week of treatment I went on a several mile walk with my wife! It's great for reversing Parkinson's symptoms!

Here are some testimonials from **Dr. Robert H. Keller's book, "Glutathione: Your Best Defense against Aging, Cellular Damage and Disease"** published in 2008.

Here is a testimonial heart problem by **Serge, 46** years old.

Back in 2005, I suffered a heart attack, three weeks before my 44th birthday. I remember thinking, "What's going on? I'm too young for this!" But it did happen. Since then, I was plagued with chronic fatigue, heart palpitation, headaches and more.

I started taking the glutathione supplement last spring and after taking it my palpitation had ceased. Then one week after my fatigue was gone and so were my headaches.

But one thing I did not expect. Since I was very young, I chewed my fingernails. (I was a nervous child) and one day, after about 3 months on the glutathione supplement, I started to notice fingernails growing for the **first time in 40 years**.

My stress levels had gone down so gradually that I did not notice that I did not chew my nails in a few days, and have not had the urge to chew my nails since then.

I've also noticed my E.D. (erectile dysfunction) as a result of my heart attack had also been corrected. My sleep patterns have also been much better, as well as my mental focus.

Glutathione patches work! J. Maggie Hardee (Myrtle Beach, S, C.)

I have been using glutathione patches since May last year. My name is Maggie Hardee. I've been in insurance sales for 15 years.

I sit in front of the computer most of my days. I do a little gardening on the side. So, I tend to hold a lot of **tension on my shoulders**.

When I started on the **glutathione patch**, I had it on my arm. Within 2 minutes, I felt like the pain on my arm just flowed out!

After 4 1/2 months of the patches, I can say my face literally feels tighter. I get more out of walking my dogs that I used to because my breathing is not as labored as it used to be.

My focus or level of clarity improved especially on the after lunch hours, 2-5PM. I wear my glutathione patches every day for 6 days. There are no side effects.
I have found my *fountain of youth*!

Suzanne Somers discusses Glutathione Patches. Check out her video testimonial.

https://www.youtube.com/watch?v=gBFTre-Y1eo

Listen to this video testimonial:

https://www.youtube.com/watch?v=U6qgniCT7Gw

One more Video Testimonial.

https://www.youtube.com/watch?v=9UyYgorfobM

Testimonials given by medical doctors who have used the product called MAX GXL from <u>www.max.com</u>

These testimonials have been collected from different sites to save you, considerable time.

Dr. Nancy Stanley

I keep myself in really good health, so I didn't feel like I needed anything to supplement my lifestyle. However, now that I've started taking Max Products, I've found that they're a great compliment to a healthy diet and exercise. I feel more energized during the day and now I'm not as tired during the afternoon.

Dr. Bryan Turner
Utah, USA

As medical director for Jordan Health and Wellness Center and a community-based hospice, Dr. Bryan Turner holds doctorates in both veterinary and human medicine (D.V.M., M.D.).

"MaxGXL has been a valuable product that many of our patients have used to **increase energy and restore health and vitality**," he says. "Most people who try it will recognize the improved well-being and see that their health begins to improve shortly after starting the capsules.

Dr. Corrine Allen
Idaho, USA

Dr. Corinne Allen is an international researcher and practitioner in natural health and nutrition and has been in practice for more than 30 years.

"I have been on MaxGXL® for four months. "My energy level has doubled."

8. Glutathione Side Effects and risks

Some side effects may occur that usually do not need medical attention. These side effects may go away during treatment as your body adjusts to the medicine. Also, your health care professional may be able to tell you about ways to prevent or reduce some of these side effects. Check with your health care professional if any of the following side effects continue or are bothersome or if you have any questions about them:

More common: Cough or hoarseness, frequent urge to defecate, straining while passing stool.

Other side effects not listed may also occur in some patients. If you notice any other effects, check with your healthcare professional. **Please read the testimonials provided earlier. One of the user had to take zinc supplements as his doctor told him "Glutathione can cause a loss of Zinc".**

Are There any Risks?

Taking glutathione as a supplement is virtually risk free however as mentioned previously, the benefits are negligible unless the glutathione is actually injected or absorbed properly by the body. Using the precursors in reasonable amounts does appear to impart worthwhile benefits but indiscriminate use of precursors such as L Cysteine are not recommended unless supervised by a health practitioner skilled in the use of specific precursors.

Glutathione ingestion and taken intravenously is contraindicated when the patient has milk protein allergies and those who may have received an organ transplant. There is no evidence to suggest that a proprietary patented blend of glutathione precursors has any contraindications in respect to the above conditions.
Although some concern does exist in regard to taking glutathione intravenously for cancer. Little or no concern is expressed when the patient can be stimulated to raise their own glutathione levels by ingesting a measured dose of precursors.

There's no evidence that supplementing with glutathione, even intravenously, is in any way going to make any cancer worse. In fact, the evidence suggests the opposite. It suggests that glutathione and other antioxidants, far from interfering with the activity of chemotherapy, appear to reduce side effects without decreasing efficacy and may, in fact, improve the efficacy of the chemotherapy in fighting cancer."

As is the norm, the experts tend to disagree on who should take glutathione or its precursors. There is no disputing the fact that glutathione levels decrease as we age so it stands to reason we should consider using the precursors to stimulate the level of glutathione in the body. Natural health advocates say everyone should take it in order to optimize their overall health. What all they acknowledge is that people with severe diseases known to be associated with low glutathione levels, may well benefit from the supplementation of precursors.

Resources

Herbs for Health and healing

http://www.amazon.com/dp/B0080UVQUU

E D T A -This Four Letter Word May Save Your Life

http://tinyurl.com/n7r7ge6

How to Prevent and Reverse Heart Diseases-and Even Avoid
By-Pass

http://tinyurl.com/k98q5b5

Pain Treatment with Magnets: Read Actual Case Histories.

http://tinyurl.com/kjcdt9e

Power of Co-Enzyme Q 10 -Health Supplements That Could Save Your Life.

http://tinyurl.com/ojvwqvr

Amazing Glutathione-Mother of All Anti-Oxidants.

http://www.amazon.com/gp/product/B00XWTX742?*Version*=1&*entries*=0

Made in United States
North Haven, CT
25 November 2024

60912350R00029